Thank You
Suzanne Somers

Gary London, M.D.

The opinions and recommendations in this book are those solely of the author. The information is not intended to be, nor should be, used as a substitute for the medical advice of other health professionals. You are advised to consult with a doctor before adopting the suggestions in this book. The author and publisher disclaim any liability arising directly or indirectly from the use of the book.

ACKNOWLEDGEMENTS

Traditionally, authors use this space to thank the people who have been of special help in the development of their books. What I have learned through the years that made it possible to write this book has been taught to me by so many educators, colleagues, patients and friends that it is impossible to thank them individually. I can only say how greatly indebted I am to each and every one of them for their contributions to my education.

I am happy, though, to be able to acknowledge three people individually. Without their encouragement, skill and editorial wisdom, this project would not have made it into this final form.

One of those is a true friend with limitless energy and extraordinary vision. Dangene McKay Bailey is a skin care expert who excels in her personal mission to help people not only look good, but also to feel good. She was quick to recognize the link between hormones and skin health and believed that more people should be aware. Her encouragement was a key motivating factor in my decision to write this book.

Another is a life-long friend. Our friendship began years before either of us even considered a career in medicine and before he became a well-known T.V. medical commentator, health educator and author. Art Ulene, M.D. has a unique talent to communicate through the written word and graciously used that talent to help me put my thoughts on paper. I deeply appreciate his unselfish efforts.

The third has been my best friend for a very long time. For many years I have described her as the smartest, wittiest, and most beautiful woman I know, but I now have to add that she is also the most skilled editor. The fact that she is also my wife only makes working on projects like this more fun and more satisfying. After a quarter century together, Joanna London often knows how to write what I am trying to say better than I can. I am grateful for her tireless work, meticulous attention to detail and boundless faith in me.

CONTENTS

GARY LONDON, M.D.
BEVERLY HILLS, CALIFORNIA

Dear Ms. Somers:

I owe you a "thank you"! Let me explain why.

People often ask me why I chose gynecology as my medical specialty. After fending off the inevitable jokes, I explain that my personal goal was simply to help women be healthy and feel their best.

Forty years in practice convinced me that I could do that for the greatest number of women by helping them delay or reverse the negative effects of aging. I had learned, as you did, that the key to maintaining or restoring vitality, beauty and sexuality was to replace the hormones that dwindle with age.

As my practice slowly evolved into one primarily focused on Natural Hormone Replacement, my greatest frustration was realizing that few women knew how easy it could be for them to take back the lives they thought were lost.

Although many books on the topic were written by brilliant and well-meaning physicians, I rarely had a patient come to me who had read one of their books or had even heard of Natural Hormone Replacement.

Then along came your book "The Sexy Years". It was so honest and clear and compelling that it introduced a huge audience to an exciting new world where vitality can outlast youth.

You are a gifted health educator, with a communication skill I admire. You have been of immeasurable help to thousands of women and to those of us who care for them.

Thank you Suzanne Somers.

Sincerely,
Gary London, M.D.

PREFACE

When I was just fifteen years old and certainly not yet planning a career, I was invited to be an observer at a birth—a very unusual opportunity for a boy of my age in the 1950's. Standing in a brightly lit, sterile room I watched in amazement as the doctor carefully guided the baby's head through an impossibly narrow passage, while at the same time calmly instructing both the mother and nurse in their roles in what certainly wasn't a calm situation. I subconsciously held my breath for a very long time while I waited for the baby to take her first gasp. Then I watched a miracle take place before my eyes as her apparently lifeless body began to move, her color turned from dark blue to pink, her eyes opened and that limp rag-doll suddenly became a normal, healthy, noisy baby.

My awe at that miraculous event (an awe that never faded even after attending over 4,500 births) was the motivation that guided me directly to my profession as an Obstetrician/ Gynecologist. Based on what I knew at the time, I thought my professional practice would be devoted primarily to helping women be safe and comfortable giving birth.

Directions of practices change, of course—sometimes because of our own experiences and sometimes because our chosen fields undergo transitions. My practice evolved through the years as I updated it so that my patients could benefit from periodic advances in the field of Women's Health Care.

I made one of my most significant changes in 1978. New information about birthing techniques at that time made many traditional procedures in labor and delivery obsolete, and I believed that it was possible to make the entire event a much more positive experience for the mother, father and even for their baby. Designing a unique physical environment and incorporating a number of advanced techniques for the birth process, I developed one of the nation's first Birth Centers. That innovative program helped to promote the concept of "gentle births" and subsequently served as a model for hospitals in redesigning their labor and delivery suites.

Several years later, my practice changed slightly when it was shown that the new technique of laparoscopic surgery had numerous advantages over traditional "open surgery" for many conditions. In order to be able to offer that advanced technique to my gynecology patients, I updated my surgical skills and added those new procedures to my practice.

Those are two examples of the many ways physicians adapt their practices to improve the health and well-being of their patients. Some changes are barely noticeable, while others might change a practice entirely.

My practice underwent another major change a few years ago when I recognized a general shift in my patients' concerns. It is a natural consequence of practicing that as a doctor ages, so do his patients. As my patients grew older, more of their complaints were about issues of physical and emotional changes that clearly resulted from aging. Helping them deal with those complaints prompted me to study the most current research and knowledge about what happens as we age.

The more I learned about aging and the essential role of Hormone Replacement Therapy in delaying or even reversing its effects, the more I came to appreciate how much the lives of my patients could be improved. Providing that therapy to an increasing number of them was very gratifying. My patients routinely and enthusiastically reported that they felt and looked better. My career had once again evolved into something I hadn't envisioned so many years ago.

Although I was pleased for my patients' success, I realized how few women, outside of practices like mine, were likely to know about this exciting new therapy. I wished that more women would learn about Natural Hormone Replacement and find a way to take advantage of the benefits it offers.

Fortunately for thousands (or perhaps millions) of women, an enlightened and courageous woman named Suzanne Somers wrote a book titled "The Sexy Years". This remarkable best-selling author, business woman and actress once again used her trusted celebrity status to improve the lives of her readers. That book was hugely successful in raising women's awareness of the benefits of Natural Hormone Replacement. Because of her work, those women are now seeking and receiving the therapy that they might otherwise have missed. The preceding letter, as well as the title of this book, is my "thank you" to her on behalf of those women and on behalf of those of us who care for them.

INTRODUCTION

This book is a condensed version of what I have learned through the years about the role that hormones play in the process of aging and the benefits of bioidentical hormones. It was written to make it as easy as possible to explain Natural Hormone Replacement and to show how it is possible to look and feel younger, be more beautiful, have more energy and vitality, increase sexuality, improve mental acuity and even live longer.

That sounds like a huge task for such a little book, doesn't it? It would take far more than these few pages if this was intended as a textbook for physicians or as a comprehensive collection of all of the relevant scientific research studies that have been done on those topics. That is not the purpose of this book. I wrote this to serve as a simple guide for my patients and others who want to know how they can retain or regain their youthful health and beauty.

When a patient comes to me for advice she doesn't want or expect me to bombard her with mountains of research material, conflicting theories and clinical studies. She expects me to teach her enough to be able to make her own intelligent decisions, but expects me, as her physician, to make recommendations. The advice I give is based upon on my training and experience gained in over four decades of study and patient care.

That is also the basis for the recommendations in this book.

I will share with you what I have learned about how you can look and feel younger. In reading this book, please consider it to be more like a consultation with a doctor than a text book. It is written the way I would talk to you in person if I had the opportunity.

The questions that make up the chapter headings are the ones I am routinely asked whenever we discuss hormone replacement. I have offered two answers for each question. The first answer is very brief, followed by a more in-depth explanation. Those of you who are satisfied with the initial short answer will be able to finish this book over your morning coffee. Those who choose to read the entire book will still find it quite easy reading, so you may be surprised when you've finished at how much you will know about your body's endocrine system, its relation to aging, and the benefits of natural hormone replacement.

This is an exciting new field of health care that challenges some long held beliefs. Determining which hormones to replenish, how much of each to prescribe and how to keep all of these hormones working in harmony is the art and science of a new medical specialty dedicated to helping you to become and remain more youthful, beautiful and vital at any age.

I.

WHAT HAPPENS AS WE AGE?

Q: *What happens as we age?*
A: *Our cells lose their ability to repair themselves when they are damaged by the normal "wear and tear" of life.*

If you are like most people, although you may intellectually accept the inevitability of aging, deep down inside you hold out the secret hope that it somehow won't happen to you. Then one day—without warning— you notice something in the mirror that is impossible to ignore. Your skin looks different, or your figure has changed. Your weight is up or your clothes don't fit. You have some body aches that you can't account for, and some leg veins you hadn't noticed before. Those dreaded telltale signs of aging seem to have suddenly appeared.

Actually, the changes in your body didn't happen suddenly. In fact, the aging process has been going on for years, beginning very subtly. While the early changes may have been subtle, the end result becomes obvious when you compare a healthy 25 year-old woman with her 75 year-old grandmother.

The vibrant, healthy young woman not only feels good, but looks good as well. She projects vitality. Her skin is moist and clear, with a youthful glow. Her muscles are toned and she moves effortlessly. She has an abundance of energy that propels her through the day without fatigue. She thinks about and enjoys sex. She sleeps well, wakes up refreshed and is anxious to enjoy the day ahead. All of her body's physiologic functions are working precisely as they were intended.

The 75 year-old presents an entirely different picture. Her skin is thin, dry, wrinkled and covered with age spots and dry patches. Her muscles are flaccid and her joints painful. Her thighs are flabby, her back hunched and her gait unsteady. She sleeps poorly and doesn't have enough energy for sex even if she were interested (which she isn't).

What happened? What caused that physical decline? And most importantly, can anything be done about it? For years, scientists around the world have asked those questions in hope that the answers would show them how to prevent aging, or at least delay it. Thanks to their research—especially breakthroughs in the last 25 years—we understand a great deal about why and how we age. We know now that the rate of aging is primarily controlled by your *endocrine system* (which also regulates your reproductive function, growth, metabolism and immune reactions). As you age, your endocrine system begins to malfunction and your body begins to fail. To understand why this happens, it helps to review how that system is intended to work.

Your body is a highly complex organism with a remarkable ability to maintain its own physiologic balance. It can do this because of constant cellular interaction and an exchange of information and nutrients back and forth from one area or system to another. Those processes are monitored and managed by an intricate network of inner intelligence. As part of that network, information is delivered to the cells of your body by *molecular messengers* which are produced by the endocrine glands. Those messengers are called "hormones" and their presence in precise amounts is necessary for your cells to do their jobs. Those jobs, including cloning themselves to heal and repair damaged tissue, are critical to your well being.

When you are young, your body can not only sense when more hormones are needed to maintain your health, but is capable of increasing hormone production as much as necessary to meet those needs. As you age, your endocrine glands begin to lose their ability to produce hormones and may not be able to keep up with your body's demands. At the same time, the aging cells throughout your body become less responsive to those hormones. Seven essential hormones that are present in abundant amounts during your youth begin to decline. That decline in hormone levels impairs your body's natural ability to repair and restore itself, because all of these hormones are involved in the feedback and repair process.

Hormone production actually begins to decline at a much earlier age than most people would associate with "aging". In fact, research shows that your hormone levels slowly start to decline after you reach your mid-twenties. At first, there may be no recognizable signs that this is occurring, because initial declines are very slight and your body is capable of adjusting to minor deficiencies. Most organs in your body have plenty of reserve capacity when you are young. However, the decline accelerates dramatically in your 40's and 50's.

Somewhere about mid-forty, give or take a few years, women have an abrupt loss of two of their essential hormones, and the effects of that drop are dramatic. Menstrual cycles are disrupted, and they begin to experience the onset of hot flashes, night sweats, insomnia, headaches, mood swings, vaginal dryness and decreased libido. That time of life, called menopause, is when ovarian function ceases. Most women are familiar with the signs and symptoms of menopause because they have either endured them themselves or have observed their mother, a sister or friends go through them. While the range and severity of those symptoms are quite variable, all women will ultimately stop having cyclic bleeding, will stop producing eggs and will no longer be able to become pregnant.

Menopause is an obvious example of the consequences of hormone deficiency. For many women it serves as a wake-up call because it provides the first clear evidence that they are actually aging. (Remember, I said earlier that even though we know better, we hold out a secret hope that it won't happen to us.) While the earlier signs were easier to ignore, the dramatic bodily changes and symptoms of menopause are not, because the ovaries shut down production of hormones so abruptly. The impact is so sudden that the episode is even nicknamed "The Change".

When other glands of the endocrine system age and become less efficient, they do so more gradually. The drop in hormone production from those glands is therefore more subtle, as are the effects. Nevertheless, activity of all of the glands diminish over time and the greater the hormone deficiency, the greater the impact. Ultimately, the reserve that protected you when you were younger is exhausted, and a "threshold" is crossed. At that point, the consequences of hormone deficiencies and imbalance become clinically evident: lean muscle mass and muscle tone decrease, body fat increases, hair gets drier and more brittle and skin gets thinner. In many people, the signs of aging include arthritic changes with joint pain, decreased energy levels, diminished brain function and increasingly troublesome loss of memory. We also begin to see a dramatic increase in the incidence of diseases such as osteoporosis and diabetes.

All of the signs and symptoms described above are evidence that normal, healthy tissue has broken down from "wear and tear". Because of age-related hormone deficiencies and imbalances, the body loses its ability to defend itself against that wear and tear.

II.

HOW CAN I STAY HEALTHY IN SPITE OF AGING?

Q: *How can I stay healthy in spite of aging?*

A: *A key step is to replace the hormones no longer being produced by your body.*

First, let me be clear about what I mean by "health". Health is much more than the absence of disease. When you are healthy, your body has firm muscles, strong bones, limber joints and radiant skin. You have a quick mind, abundant energy and a vibrant sexuality. The 75 year-old woman described in the previous chapter has none of those characteristics. She is not healthy, but neither is she diseased. She is debilitated by age. Her body can no longer repair and heal itself as it did when she was young, because she no longer has an adequate amount of the essential hormones that were circulating through her body at peak levels when she was 25 years old.

The cells and organs in your body are born with a remarkable ability to heal themselves—not only from the effects of physical injury, but also from the normal wear and tear of daily life. A good example of this is what happens when you cut your finger. As it heals, the skin restores all of its layers perfectly and resumes its original appearance. It even reproduces your unique fingerprints. Some major organs like the liver are able to regenerate themselves and resume normal function after a large portion has been removed surgically.

Imagine how convenient it would be if your car's tires could restore themselves from the wear and tear of driving while the car rested in the garage each night, or if the logs in your fireplace could heal themselves after you burned them? As far-fetched as those fantasy examples sound, that's exactly what your body does when it recovers from injury or it repairs the effects of aging.

Every system in your body is designed to maintain as perfect a state of health as possible. It accomplishes this through a remarkable set of "feed-back" systems that monitor and balance each and every function, down to the tiniest intracellular biochemical reaction. An infinite number of complex processes are going on in your body at all times. They all rely on hormones for intercellular communication, as described in the previous chapter. You are dependent upon many different hormones, each with unique functions. A deficiency in any of those hormones results in diminished functions of the cells it is designed to target.

Your body has ways to communicate with you when it detects a deficiency in any essential element. For example, when it needs fuel, your body signals you with a sensation you recognize as hunger. When its sensors detect a negative balance of water in its cells, it signals you with a sensation you recognize as thirst. Those are obvious and bold messages, but only two of thousands of equally important messages being sent continuously throughout your body in its effort to maintain health and physiologic balance. Signs and symptoms of aging are your body's messages to you that your hormones are deficient.

So, what—if anything—can you do about it? Must your health decline because your hormone levels are falling? Are the ravages of age inevitable? Thanks to scientists who have taken on the challenge of combating aging, we are no longer helpless in dealing with this problem. Research shows that it is possible to prevent or delay the downward spiral associated with aging. Prevention is, of course, the best way to deal with any negative event, and aging is no exception. By identifying when your hormone levels begin to decline and measuring exactly how much they have dropped, we can now replace the missing hormones and prevent that progressive deterioration.

Even if damage has already occurred, we can now reverse much of it by restoring diminished hormones to *optimum* levels. (Optimum levels are the amount of hormones that were circulating in your blood when you were 25 years old and at your peak of health and performance.)

This is not to suggest that hormone replacement will keep you permanently at one age. You will still continue to age and lose cells based upon a cellular life cycle that is genetically determined. Each cell in your body can replicate only so many times until it runs out of genetic material.

The goal of hormone replacement is not to live forever, but to avoid the precipitous decline that begins about age 40. I believe it is possible to live in excellent health, with vitality and resiliency for many more years by replenishing the hormones that occur naturally in our bodies to optimum, medically sound levels.

III.

WHAT IS A HORMONE?

Q: *What is a hormone?*

A: *A substance produced by a gland and transported in the bloodstream throughout the body, transferring informa-tion and instructions between cells.*

The definition above is factually correct, but still leaves most people confused about what hormones really are, where they come from, and what they do. In order to appreciate the expla-nation of replacement therapy in a later chapter, it is important that you have a clear understanding of hormones.

Hormones are molecules that are synthesized and secreted by several glands throughout the body, collectively known as the endocrine system. The primary glands of that system include the adrenals (which are perched on top of the kidneys), the testes (in the male scrotum), the ovaries (located in the female pelvis, one on each side of the uterus), the pancreas (located in the abdomen, just beneath the diaphragm), the thyroid (found in the front of the neck), and the pituitary (in the skull).

Each gland produces its own unique hormones, and each of those hormones serves as a molecular messenger to deliver very specific information to specific cells or organs in the body. Almost like a key opening a lock, these hormones have the abil-ity to turn certain cells in the body (known as target cells) "on" and "off". Each hormone has its own specific target cells (for example, there are specific target cells in the breast and uterus that will respond to estrogen), and each target cell is genetically programmed to respond to particular hormones in a certain way. All aspects of cellular function, including repair and repli-cation, are influenced by one or more hormones.

The process of achieving and maintaining true health

involves many hormones at the same time, with all of their levels continually adjusting to the constant changes your body is experiencing. Thanks to the sensitive feed-back mechanisms I described earlier, a delicate balance is maintained between all of the hormones in your body. To maintain this balance, your body must produce greater or lesser amounts of each hormone at different times of the day, month, and stage of life. Some of these variations are designed to control normal physiologic functions. An example would be the cyclic changes in ovarian hormones that regulate your menstrual periods. Those cyclic variations are healthy and are necessary for reproduction. Other variations, caused by glandular failure, are detrimental to your health. Menopause (which occurs when your ovaries fail) is an example of this.

The ovaries are not the only glands that wear out with aging. In fact, all glands begin to wear out and become less efficient in their production of hormones. Research shows that replacing the missing hormones—if done properly—can help you maintain your physiological equilibrium and prevent the consequences of hormonal failure. In the next chapter, I'll show you which hormones are of primary concern, and tell you why.

IV.

WHICH HORMONES SHOULD I BE CONCERNED ABOUT?

Q: *Which hormones should I be concerned about?*

A: *The seven major hormones that are necessary for a woman to remain youthful, vibrant and healthy are: estrogen, progesterone, testosterone, thyroid, DHEA, pregnenolone and HGH.*

In any discussion about hormones, most women immediately think about estrogen and progesterone. Those two have always received the most attention in regard to women's health issues. Actually, there are *seven* major hormones that are necessary for you to remain youthful, vibrant and healthy. Each one produces unique, distinct and independent effects that contribute to your overall well-being. However, all hormones must work together in perfect balance to achieve their maximum effectiveness. This is true at any age, not just in the years of decline. The goal of natural hormone therapy is to keep these seven essential hormones at the optimum level and in perfect balance for as long as possible.

What follows in the next few pages is a much abbreviated review of these seven key hormones with an explanation of their functions. There have been entire books written on each of these hormones, so this is in no way intended to be a comprehensive review. I believe, nonetheless, that you will find enough information to appreciate the essential role each one plays in your life and health.

THANK YOU SUZANNE SOMERS / 31

ESTROGEN

There are three types of estrogen found in a woman's body, each with a slightly different molecular structure: estrone, estradiol and estriol. These estrogens, which are produced primarily in the ovaries and, to a lesser extent in the adrenal glands, are usually considered together as "estrogen".

Estrogen is the hormone that initiates the physical transformation from childhood to womanhood. It is responsible for all of the physical characteristics that we associate with femininity including development of the breasts and lubrication of the vagina. During the reproductive years, estrogen helps create the proper environment in the uterus for implantation and nourishment of the early embryo. Estrogen has some very beneficial functions beyond the reproductive tract. For instance, it reacts with the endorphins in the brain to enhance a feeling of well-being. Also, it plays an important role in preserving the youthful appearance and texture of your skin, by maintaining its elasticity and promoting the retention of moisture.

For much of your life, estrogen levels fluctuate up and down. This occurs not only at the beginning and end of each menstrual cycle, but throughout the month as well. The levels also depend on the stage of your life. The amount of estrogen produced falls dramatically at the onset of menopause and even more precipitously if the ovaries are surgically removed before the natural onset of menopause. The resulting deficiency in estrogen causes symptoms such as hot flashes, night sweats, insomnia, vaginal dryness, bladder problems, difficulty concentrating and emotional instability. The risk of certain disease processes, including osteoporosis, heart disease, stroke, and

Alzheimer's disease also increases in the absence of estrogen. Problems caused by estrogen deficiency have been recognized for a very long time, and estrogen, in a variety of forms, has been used for almost half a century to relieve menopausal symptoms and to treat estrogen-deficiency disorders. There is no doubt that estrogen can protect against many of the effects of aging, including wrinkled and dry skin, sagging breasts, fatigue, depression, mood swings and decreased libido. However, as with all other drugs and medications, estrogen only works if the right form is chosen and prescribed in the proper amount at the appropriate time. As a practicing physician, I am ever mindful of the ongoing challenge involved in making sure those criteria are met.

Later in this book I will discuss some of the specific challenges related to estrogen use (for example: the issue of "natural" versus synthetic hormones). For now, I'll simply summarize the conclusions I've reached after reviewing the scientific literature and working with patients for more than forty years: When estrogen levels decline, this hormone should be replaced with a natural hormone that is biochemically identical to the estrogen produced by the human body. It should be replaced in sufficient amounts to maintain the optimum level, and its use should be closely monitored.

PROGESTERONE

Progesterone is a female hormone produced by the ovaries and adrenal glands. Because of its many important functions in women, it should probably share equal billing with estrogen, but it is not nearly as well known. It plays a critical role in procreation, by preparing the cells that line the uterus so they are ready to receive and sustain a pregnancy. Another of its primary functions is to *balance* the effects of estrogen, preventing a potentially damaging effect that can occur when estrogen is present alone. Progesterone also helps to strengthen bones. It relieves menopausal symptoms and decreases headaches, bloating, irritability, and moodiness associated with menstruation and PMS.

A woman produces very little progesterone until she begins ovulating (producing eggs for reproduction). Beginning at that stage of her life, progesterone is produced in significant amounts only during the last two weeks of her four-week cycle. When ovulation occurs (at about 14 days in a woman who is having 28-day cycles), the ovary begins to produce large amounts of progesterone. The level of progesterone in the body peaks about one week later, and then falls if fertilization has not taken place. (If an egg has been fertilized and a pregnancy begins, progesterone production will increase dramatically in order to support the pregnancy.)

Progesterone production begins to slow when a woman is in her thirties, and declines rapidly during her forties. By age 45 to 50, when ovulation has ceased to occur in almost all women, progesterone deficiency is virtually universal. All women are progesterone deficient in menopause. The scant amounts produced at that time are not sufficient to perform this hormone's many physiologic tasks.

The drop in progesterone levels actually starts earlier and occurs more rapidly than the decline of estrogen. Because of this early decline, insufficient progesterone is available for its important function of counterbalancing the estrogen that is present. This results in a condition known as "estrogen dominance", a root cause of many female problems, including irregular periods, heavy bleeding and endometrial polyps. Estrogen dominance also complicates adenomyosis and endometriosis (two conditions related to uterine disorders) and is responsible for the troublesome complaints of bloating and breast tenderness.

Restoring progesterone to an optimum level makes it easier to manage the conditions listed above. This hormone has many other benefits: it acts as a diuretic, helping the body rid itself of excess retained water; it produces a calming, anti-anxiety effect; enhances your body's defenses; improves breakdown of fat into energy; cuts the craving for carbohydrates and sweets; reduces breast tenderness and contributes to the formation of new bone tissue.

Until recently, most women who have been treated with "progesterone" were actually receiving one of several synthetic chemicals known as *progestins*, which were thought to duplicate the functions of the naturally occurring progesterone. However, the receptor sites on human cells are genetically programmed to recognize and accept the molecular structure of natural progesterone, and not synthetic analogs. Consequently those synthetic products can cause side effects and are potentially harmful. The proper substance to use for restoring progesterone to optimum levels is a natural hormone that is biochemically identical ("bioidentical") to the one produced by your body.

TESTOSTERONE

Even though testosterone is known primarily as a male hormone, it is also produced in a woman's ovaries and adrenal glands, and adequate amounts of this hormone are crucial to her well being. Women need far less testosterone than men, so the ovaries produce far less than do men's testes, and less of this hormone is needed for restoration to proper levels.

As in the male, testosterone is responsible for a woman's sex drive. It is the motivating force that increases libido, enhances mood and improves sexual performance. For any woman who feels that her sexuality is fading, those would be reasons enough to want her testosterone boosted, but this hormone has many other critical functions.

Testosterone plays a major role in building muscle mass, strength and tone, while simultaneously decreasing stored fat. That combination gives your figure more youthful definition. This hormone also elevates your energy level and your enthusiasm for exercise while improving your endurance. Testosterone is also known to improve skin tone and prevent wrinkles by increasing the amount of collagen in skin. Additionally, it aids your body's capacity to heal, enhances your memory, and protects against the development of Alzheimer's disease.

In young women, testosterone helps develop stamina, stronger muscles and feelings of strength and security. By age thirty-five, there is a substantial decrease in testosterone production by women, with an accompanying decline in these traits. Soon thereafter, women begin to notice a decrease in skin tightness. This is partially because the muscles beneath the skin are losing their size and firmness, leaving the skin saggy.

Another important benefit of testosterone is its contribution to increased bone density and prevention of osteoporosis. Our bones are constantly being renewed cellularly, but that process requires hormones which enable your body to incorporate building materials like calcium. You have seen how elderly women shrink in height and how their backs curve from collapse of their spinal vertebrae. This is graphic evidence of the damage caused by osteoporosis resulting from inadequate hormones. Most women are familiar with the preventive value of estrogen replacement therapy, but few are aware of the additional value of testosterone in preventing bone loss.

Around the time of menopause, testosterone levels continue to drop, but not as rapidly as estrogen levels. This disrupts the delicate balance that existed between these two hormones, and creates the possibility of testosterone dominance. In this situation, even though testosterone levels are lower than before, signs of testosterone *excess* may occur, such as acne and unwanted hair growth. This is the reason why it is important to monitor not only the levels of all hormones, but also to consider the balance between them.

In order to restore peak physical and mental performance, every hormone must be restored to its optimum level, and the balance maintained with other hormones. Both actions are particularly important with testosterone.

THYROID

Thyroid hormone, secreted by the thyroid gland in the neck, regulates temperature, metabolism, and certain brain functions. To appreciate the importance of this hormone, it's helpful to look at what happens to your body when it is lacking. Low thyroid (technically known as "hypothyroidism") causes weight gain, fatigue, depression, forgetfulness, dry skin, brittle fingernails, thin hair, sleep disturbance and lethargy. When these symptoms are observed in a young person, they are likely to be identified as signs of hypothyroidism and be appropriately treated. In an older person, however, they are often dismissed as normal signs of aging. Fortunately, with simple blood tests, thyroid hormone deficiency can be easily identified and treated.

Thyroid is one of my favorite hormones, because results from replacement therapy are often so dramatic and gratifying. This is especially true when it comes to weight gain. One of the most frequent complaints from my 40-something patients is that, in spite of rigid dieting and compulsive exercise, they not only can't lose weight, but may be gaining. If testing confirms a deficiency in thyroid (and it often does), then within weeks of treatment these women begin to enjoy the weight loss that had been so elusive. Thyroid hormone increases fat breakdown and lowers blood cholesterol levels. It increases energy and mental alertness and decreases forgetfulness and mental confusion. It supports a healthy immune system, and relieves symptoms of thin hair, dry skin and brittle nails.

Two forms of thyroid hormone are found in the body, and it is important to recognize the difference between them. The form produced by the thyroid gland is a storage form called T-4. Once that storage form makes its way into the blood stream, it is converted by a special enzyme to the active form, called T-3. As we age, we not only tend to produce less thyroid hormone, just as we produce less of our other hormones, but our ability to convert it to T-3 also declines. Compounding the problem, the target cells that thyroid hormone is programmed to stimulate become less efficient in their ability to respond. These factors combine, resulting in the symptoms described above.

Fortunately, restoring thyroid to an optimum level can correct these symptoms. Often, when someone who has been deficient in thyroid begins replacement therapy, improvements are so dramatic that they are obvious not only to the patient, but to everyone around her.

In order to assess your needs for thyroid replacement, it is necessary to measure the thyroid hormone in your blood. If a deficiency is detected, replacement should be with a compounded natural thyroid that includes both T-3 and T-4. Synthetic thyroid products containing only T-4 are not as effective, and do not seem to be as well metabolized or tolerated.

DHEA

DHEA is an abbreviation for "dehydroepiandrosterone", a hormone produced primarily by the adrenal glands. It is called a "precursor" because the body converts it to estrogen and testosterone. Additionally, DHEA also has its own important functions. At this time, there are literally thousands of published scientific reports documenting the benefits of this hormone.

DHEA has become the darling of the supplement and antiaging community because of scientific studies which show that patients who use this hormone sleep better, have more energy, and handle stress better. DHEA acts as a mood elevator, improves the function of the immune system and improves brain function. It is known to decrease insulin resistance which improves the utilization of blood sugar for energy and helps prevent diabetes. When DHEA was given to women who were not responding to fertility drugs, their response to these medications improved dramatically.

As with so many other hormones, your body's production of DHEA peaks around the age of twenty-five (when we are also at our lifetime peak of health and vitality). It then declines with the passage of time. By age fifty, we are producing only half as much DHEA and some elderly people produce none at all. A deficiency in DHEA is associated with lack of stamina, fatigue, stress, decreased immunity, memory loss, dry skin, and poor sex drive.

DHEA is an important element in any comprehensive hormone replacement program. This hormone is not a prescription item, and can be purchased from numerous sources. Unfortunately, the purity and strength of those products is often questionable. Also, the duration of action of over-the-counter DHEA is so short that you would have to take it three times a day to maintain an optimum level. If you plan to supplement your body with DHEA, you should use a pure pharmaceutical grade that is prepared by a compounding pharmacy in a micronized, sustained-release form.

PREGNENOLONE

Pregnenolone is produced by the adrenal gland and brain. Like DHEA, it is called a precursor because of its role in the production of other hormones. Pregnenolone is metabolized into progesterone and DHEA, which are in turn transformed into other hormones.

Pregnenolone plays a subtle and supportive role in the body's physiology. Highest levels of pregnenolone are found in the brain, where it aids in cell repair and brain function. Like other hormones, its production declines with age. By forty, we have half the amount we had at age 20. When pregnenolone drops, so does the production of other hormones in the steroid pathway.

Research suggests that pregnenolone could be the most potent memory enhancer of all time. Studies show that it can contribute to enhanced alertness, increased learning ability and intelligence. Pregnenolone promotes feelings of well-being, helps reduce the emotional symptoms of PMS and is considered an anti-stress hormone. Patients with rheumatoid arthritis reported that they had less pain and fatigue when they were treated with pregnenolone.

As with DHEA, pregnenolone should be prescribed in a micronized sustained-release form, prepared by a compounding pharmacy using pure pharmaceutical grade hormone.

HUMAN GROWTH HORMONE

The name "human growth hormone" (HGH) is misleading, because it gives the false impression that it will make things grow at what could be an inappropriate time of life. In fact, this hormone does promote physical growth, but only during childhood. In mature adults, HGH is a healing hormone with powerful anti-aging benefits, and it has already proven its value in promoting vitality and youthfulness.

HGH is produced by the pituitary gland in the brain. After its release into the bloodstream, it promotes healing throughout the body by stimulating cell growth and rejuvenation. Optimum levels of this hormone are associated with low body fat and cholesterol, good muscle tone, youthful elasticity of skin, healthy immune function, mental clarity, high energy and mental well-being.

Like other hormones, HGH peaks in our early twenties and then begins to decline. By age fifty, levels of HGH have dropped to half of their peak, and production continues on a downward slide thereafter.

The effects of declining HGH are evident in signs such as loss of skin elasticity. The skin becomes thinner, and is easily separated from the underlying tissue. (Gently pinch the skin on the back of your hand and pull it upward. If it returns slowly, that is a sign of aging skin.) Other signs of HGH deficiency include increased body fat, decreased lean muscle mass, loss of bone density, poor sleep, thinning hair, and lower metabolic rate.

Many studies have shown that replenishing low levels of HGH can delay and even reverse the aging process, and return patients to a more vigorous state of health. Striking evidence of its ability to reverse the aging process was demonstrated when a group of men in their 50's and 60's was treated with HGH. Their abdominal fat decreased and their lean muscle mass increased—just the opposite from what is usually seen at that age. When used before and after surgery, HGH greatly enhances post-operative healing. For that reason, it is used by many plastic surgeons who are striving for the best possible cosmetic results.

HGH offers tremendous benefits for people who exercise. This hormone enhances exercise capacity, increases endurance and strength, and improves recovery after intense exercise. As we pass through our 40's, an almost universal complaint of men (and to a lesser extent, women) is that their muscles stop responding to exercise. Before then, an hour workout with weights was rewarded with larger, firmer, more defined muscles. As we age, those heavy-duty workouts no longer seem to produce the same results. The reason: we don't have adequate amounts of the hormones necessary to trigger growth of muscle cells. HGH is one of those key hormones.

In spite of the benefits provided by HGH, many people are initially reluctant to try it when they learn that the only effective way to raise HGH to therapeutic levels is through daily self-administered injections of the hormone—exactly the same way that people with diabetes take their insulin. That may sound frightening, but there really is little or no discomfort, thanks to the very fine needles that are now available. In fact, the pain of injections may be far easier to tolerate than the cost, because injectable HGH is quite costly. Fortunately, that is beginning to change, thanks to genetic engineering advances that are making increased production possible. (This is the same technology used to produce insulin today.) Although still expensive, injectable HGH is no longer out of reach for those who appreciate the benefits it offers. In my opinion, HGH may be the closest we have yet come to a "fountain of youth".

Don't be fooled by the false promises of those who promote worthless products—like "oral growth hormone"—that claim to be as effective as the injectable form of HGH. These claims for over-the-counter and network marketing products are based on studies that actually used injectable growth hormone. There is no evidence that the oral products (which the promoters call "secretagogues") have any significant effect, or that they are at all comparable to injectable HGH. To get any benefit from HGH restoration, you must use pure injectable hormone prescribed by a physician and supplied by a reputable pharmaceutical company.

* * *

Individually, each of the hormones I have just described is essential to your health. Their *collective* activity is even more important. Years of research and clinical studies have clearly proven that estrogen, progesterone, testosterone, thyroid, DHEA, pregnenolone and HGH must *all* be present in carefully balanced levels for you to remain youthful and healthy.

V.

ARE "NATURAL" HORMONES BETTER?

Q: *Are "natural" hormones better?*
A: *Yes.*

Natural hormones are better for you than the synthetic products that claim to give the same results. This is because of their molecular structure, not where they come from or how they are manufactured.

Every substance has a unique chemical formula and all of its molecular elements are arranged in a specific pattern. That specific configuration is known as its *molecular structure*. A "natural" hormone is one whose molecular structure is identical to that of the hormone produced by the glands in your body. We call that "bioidentical". A synthetic hormone, such as Premarin or Provera, although designed to mimic the actions of your body's hormones as much as possible, has a different molecular structure than your body's own.

The reason that synthetic hormones are produced and have been used so extensively for so many years is due to the economics of the pharmaceutical industry. Research, testing, government approvals and marketing are all enormously expensive. It takes hundreds of millions of dollars to bring a new drug to market. The only way a drug company can afford to make such an enormous investment is to insure that it has the exclusive right to sell the newly invented drug for many years, allowing it to recoup its investment and make a profit. The way it insures its exclusivity is to secure a patent on the new drug which prevents competitors from selling a copy-cat drug. That is the way all new drugs reach the market, and it is this profit potential that can be credited with the development of the many miraculous drugs and medications available to us.

Major drug companies wanted products to sell that could treat symptoms of hormone deficiency, regulate menses and provide contraception. Because no one is allowed to secure a patent on a bioidentical or natural hormone, the drug companies created synthetic hormones that could be patented. Those hormones are intended to produce the same results as your body's own, but the molecular structures of those synthetic products are different.

Synthetic drugs also have different risks of side effects and complications. Several large research projects recently reported that long-term use of synthetic hormones increased certain health risks. Unfortunately, the widely publicized results of those studies frightened many women (and their doctors) into abandoning hormone replacement therapy completely. This is one of the reasons for so much current interest in natural hormone replacement therapy.

Your body is able to utilize natural hormones more efficiently than synthetics because their molecular structure is identical to your body's own hormones. Target cells throughout your body have been genetically programmed to respond to those particular molecules. Because synthetic compounds are not metabolized in the same way as natural hormones, they leave waste products and produce unwanted side-effects.

Unfortunately, little research has been done that directly compares the long-term risks and benefits of natural hormones versus synthetics. This is primarily because natural hormones can not be patented, so there is no financial incentive for any pharmaceutical company to prove their value. However, there are numerous articles in the scientific literature identifying significant differences in side effects when using the two types.

This is especially true of well-tolerated natural progesterone as compared to the synthetic progestins which cause fluid retention, bloating, headaches and depression. Estrogen side-effects are also minimized with bioidentical hormone, and a combination of natural estrogen with natural progesterone has been shown to result in an improved lipid profile over synthetics. Thyroid is another hormone that seems to have better effectiveness and be more easily tolerated in its natural form.

It's only logical that your body will perform better and be less likely to suffer negative side-effects when it is exposed to elements that were included in its original genetic design. That's why you feel better when your deficient hormones are replaced with exact replicas of the originals.

After studying the available literature and considering the collective wisdom of the experts in this field whose judgment I trust, there is no question in my mind about the choice between natural hormones and synthetic. Natural is better.

VI.

WHO NEEDS REPLACEMENT HORMONES?

Q: *Who needs replacement hormones?*

A: *If you are over 40, you probably do. And even if you are under 40, but have no energy, or trouble maintaining your weight, or have irregular periods, or no interest in sex, you probably do.*

If you have been going through this book chapter by chapter, you have read several times that your hormones begin to decline as early as your mid-twenties. That doesn't mean that you should start replacing them at such a young age. Minor changes are not harmful, and your body is perfectly capable of adjusting to slight reductions without suffering any damage. By 40, however, some people are experiencing symptoms caused by that decline that are hard to ignore. To illustrate that point, consider the complaints of three of my patients.

Madeline G. is a 41 year old mother of three who has never had to worry much about her weight. She has always eaten sensibly, exercised only occasionally, and enjoyed what most people would consider a very attractive figure. Suddenly, in the last two years, without changing her diet or her physical activity, Madeline has gained 12 pounds and two dress sizes. Troubled, she started watching her diet and joined a gym. In spite of giving up several of her favorite foods and working out three mornings a week, her weight hasn't dropped an ounce, and she still can't wear half of the clothes in her closet.

Lois W. is 49 years old, and had normal menstrual cycles every month from age 16 to 48, except when she was pregnant. For the last year, however, her bleeding has been totally irregular. She never knows when to expect a period, how long it will last, or how heavy it will be. She occasionally skips a month or two, and sometimes bleeds for as many as 12 days in a month. Betty R. is 61. She went through menopause at age 54, and endured months of hot flashes, sweats and mood swings before her doctor prescribed Premarin. Most of her menopausal symptoms have cleared, and she hasn't bled for years. Now, however, she has a new set of troubling symptoms. Her muscles are becoming flabby. She is gaining weight, and it all is accumulating around her stomach, hips and thighs. Her skin is thinner and looser, her energy is low, and her interest in sex is even lower. She doesn't sleep well, and wakes up tired and achy. Most troubling of all is her failing memory. She sometimes has difficulty remembering even the most basic things like her address or what she planned to pick up at the market once she gets there.

At first glance, these patients might seem to have unrelated problems, but their examinations and testing showed that they all had one thing in common: a hormone deficiency or imbalance. These cases show some of the variation in the ways that hormone deficiency manifests itself. The differences occur because these women differ in age, genetic makeup, body type and life style as well as the presence or absence of other health conditions. Symptoms also depend on which specific hormones a woman is lacking.

Do you recognize yourself in any of these stories? Do some of those complaints sound familiar? If you are over 40, chances are good that you do because all women go through the same biological changes over time. If you are lucky, your symptoms may come later than your friends', or may not be as troublesome. But, sooner or later, you are sure to be affected. If you are not happy with that prospect, you should consider doing something to alter that otherwise inevitable course.

Taking action is not difficult, but does require that your hormone deficiencies be identified and corrected. Nobody can turn back the clock and make you 25 years old again, but—no matter what your age—restoring hormone function offers a number of benefits. It can help you look more beautiful, increase your energy, improve your sex life and sleep better. It can help you manage your weight more easily, control menopausal symptoms and regulate or eliminate bleeding. In general, it can help you enjoy a more vital, satisfying life.

VII.

WILL I LOOK BETTER?

Q: *Will I look better?*

A: *Yes. You will look younger, healthier and more beautiful.*

Did I get your attention with that answer? Let me explain why I am willing to make such a bold promise.

Whenever we look at someone, we tend to judge their age, health and beauty using an arbitrary set of criteria. Consciously or subconsciously, we go through that process each and every time we come in contact with another person. Although any two of us may disagree on which criteria to use in our "judging" or on the exact ranking of a particular person (remember, beauty is in the eye of the beholder), we all judge the same features. Everyone looks at skin, muscle, adipose tissue, posture, body motion and energy. These features are important to almost all of us when we categorize someone as young or old, healthy or unhealthy, beautiful or not.

Skin is especially easy to evaluate because the changes over time are so recognizable. Young, healthy skin is soft, smooth and thick with good color and elasticity. With aging it becomes dry, thin, wrinkled and saggy and it loses its elasticity. Overall, the appearance of your skin is one of the most readily visible signs of aging. Fortunately, those negative changes in your skin can be delayed or reversed with supplemental hormones.

Estrogen increases collagen and retains moisture in the inner layer of skin. This supports the outer layer, providing more elasticity and firmness while decreasing sagging. *Testosterone* also increases collagen which improves skin tone and prevents wrinkles. Low *thyroid* contributes to dry skin (and also makes nails brittle and hair thin). These signs of aging can be avoided or corrected by restoring thyroid to normal levels. A deficiency in

DHEA is also associated with dry skin, while thinning of the skin and loss of elasticity are caused by declining *HGH*. Replacing these two hormones helps to correct these problems. Hormones play another important role when it comes to your skin. They will help you get better results from your skin treatments. For example, microdermabrasion and facial peels remove superficial dead skin and expose the newer, healthier cells below. Your skin will heal and respond best when your hormones are at their optimum levels. The same is true for LED Light Therapy. That new innovation prompts the skin's fibroblasts to produce collagen and proteins deep within the skin. Cells kept healthy with youthful levels of hormones are best able to perform those functions. Even bleaching creams and moisturizers work better on healthy skin. Skin is very responsive to replacement therapy. If your skin is showing the effects of hormone deficiencies, you can expect to see marked improvement as hormones are replenished to optimum levels. With improved skin, you will *look* better.

The ratio of lean muscle mass to body fat is another measure of youth, health and beauty. Some of us are more attracted to leaner body types while others prefer bulkier bodies, but we all appreciate firm, toned muscles and almost all agree that there is a limit to the amount of fat that is attractive or looks healthy. Testosterone is primarily responsible for building muscle mass, while decreasing stored fat. Testosterone also raises your level of energy and improves exercise endurance. Without this hormone it is difficult, if not impossible, for you to maintain an attractive figure with youthful definition.

Uncontrollable weight gain, one of the most common complaints of aging, is often caused by low levels of thyroid. Once this problem has been identified and corrected, weight management becomes much easier.

A well documented research study showed that HGH increased lean muscle mass and reduced abdominal fat. It has also been shown to increase endurance and strength. Maintaining all of these hormones at proper levels will help you have a leaner, more toned and sculpted body. You will look better.

I also mentioned posture as a feature that we tend to consider in our evaluation of others. Posture is partially dependent upon muscle tone and discipline, but not entirely. The strength of your bones is another significant factor in your ability to stand tall and straight. Unfortunately, osteoporosis (the so-called brittle bone disease), is a common complication of aging. The rapid loss of bone mass seen after menopause is due to the declining levels of estrogen. This results in thinner, more brittle bones that are much more likely to fracture. One of the consequences, collapse of the spinal vertebrae, is ultimately responsible for the shrinking height and hunching over we see in older women. Estrogen is widely accepted as treatment for osteoporosis and is very effective.

Progesterone also contributes to the formation of new bone, as does testosterone. HGH has the ability to defend against bone loss as well. Testosterone and HGH both help maintain healthy joints, which are required for good posture. When your muscles and joints are strong, flexible and pain free, your body moves fluidly and gracefully. With good posture and graceful body motion, you will look better.

Finally, it's important to remind you of the energy-enhancing power of all seven hormones that I discussed earlier in this book. Estrogen protects against fatigue and depression and enhances a feeling of well-being. Progesterone decreases moodiness. Testosterone elevates energy level, increases enthusiasm for exercise and promotes stamina. Thyroid hormone combats fatigue and lethargy. Studies on DHEA showed that patients receiving it had more energy. Pregnenolone, in addition to its important role as a precursor to other hormones, has its own functions of contributing to alertness and decreasing stress. Last, but not least, is HGH which is a potent factor in maintaining high energy. Each of these seven hormones has a role in enhancing your energy and vitality, both of which will definitely help you look better.

For all of the above reasons, I stand by my claim that you will look better if you maintain your essential hormones at optimum levels. The features that other people will use to evaluate your age, health and beauty are all enhanced by those hormones. With better appearing skin, firmer muscles, less body fat, good posture and high energy you will look younger, healthier and more beautiful.

VIII.

WILL SEX IMPROVE?

Q: *Will sex improve?*
A: *Yes, for many reasons.*

The desire to improve sex is one of the primary forces driving people to seek hormone therapy, because of a widely held belief (or at least hope) that sexual dissatisfaction can be cured with hormones. In many cases, hormone deficiency is the major problem. However, it is important to note that many other factors including stress, fatigue, general health, and relationships also greatly influence the quality of your sex life.

When discussing sex, there are three basic elements that should be considered: desire, performance and satisfaction. Let's look at each of these in greater detail.

DESIRE

A simplified definition of *desire* is "the interest in being sexual". That interest may arise spontaneously from within, or it can arise in response to a partner's words or actions. This interest or desire is usually referred to as *libido*. There is general agreement that testosterone plays a critical role in producing an active libido in both women and men. Studies have correlated low testosterone levels in both sexes with low sexual desire. It's not surprising therefore, that when libido begins to decline, the problem is often caused by a drop in testosterone.

Research shows that testosterone levels in women in their 40's are half the levels of women in their 20's. A similar decline is seen in the levels of DHEA, the primary precursor to testosterone. DHEA peaks at age 25, slips to half of that level by age

50, and may be totally absent in the elderly. (Remember, since DHEA is a precursor to testosterone, any reduction in DHEA results in lower testosterone levels.)

Replacing testosterone is a key step in improving a woman's libido, and it has been proven to be greatly successful in doing so. In my practice, numerous patients (and their happy partners) attest to the remarkable improvement they have enjoyed following use of testosterone.

PERFORMANCE

The second key sexual element to consider is *performance*—one aspect of which is physical activity. It is not necessary to be a "sexual athlete" to have a fully satisfying sex life, but it certainly helps to have a reasonable amount of strength, energy and endurance. Both testosterone and HGH build muscle mass, boost energy, and improve exercise endurance. That's why restoring these two hormones to their optimum levels will improve your sexual performance.

Testosterone plays another important role in sexual performance by increasing genital blood flow, which increases the sensitivity and responsiveness of the clitoris. Re-awakening a sleeping clitoris is certain to enhance performance.

Performance is also highly dependent upon the health of a woman's vagina, which in turn depends on adequate amounts of estrogen. Low estrogen levels decrease vaginal lubrication and thin the vaginal lining, which result in vaginal dryness, itching, burning and pain with penetration. Low levels of estrogen also reduce vaginal blood flow and impede nerve transmission, which impair sexual function. Replacement estrogen is highly effective in treating these problems.

SATISFACTION

The third sexual element, *satisfaction,* is the most difficult to address, because the term is so ambiguous. Failure to be "satisfied" means different things to different people. For some women, it means failure to achieve orgasm. For others it can refer to inadequate frequency of sex or diminished libido. Still others would cite entirely different problems. Medical researchers have attempted to classify unsatisfactory sex life with terms such as Female Sexual Dysfunction (FSD) and Hypoactive Sexual Desire Disorder (HSDD).

Using the criteria established by some experts, 40-50% of all women would be classified as having a "sexual disorder". Whether or not the criteria for classifying sexual disorders are valid, surveys of women make one thing clear: for a large percentage of them, their sex life is not entirely satisfactory. Many reasons are given for the dissatisfaction, and not all are related to hormones. Nevertheless, hormone deficiencies are responsible for many of their complaints, and in those cases, the problems are best solved by replacing deficient hormones and maintaining them at optimum levels.

Let's review why hormone replacement works for so many women. The seven essential hormones are known to increase libido, increase vaginal blood flow, increase vaginal lubrication, increase sensitivity of the clitoris, improve muscle tone, reduce body fat and weight, improve endurance, elevate energy, enhance mood, relieve menopausal symptoms, decrease depression, relieve fatigue, decrease headaches and relieve stress. Any one of these important actions could be expected to result in improved sex. Combine several of them, and there's likely to be a major improvement that any woman will appreciate.

The importance of sexual desire, performance and satisfaction is something each person must decide for herself. Some facts, however, are universal: healthy people are more sexual and sexual people are healthier; and, when a woman's sex life is satisfying, she feels more feminine, more attractive and more alive. Hormones are essential to achieving this.

IX.

ARE THE BENEFITS
WORTH THE RISKS?

Q. Are the benefits worth the risks?

A. In my opinion, yes. After considering the facts, you get to make your own final decision.

The issue of risks always generates the most debate when hormones are being discussed. There are risks, of course, in almost everything we do in life, and we are constantly making decisions about which risks we are willing to take and which ones we want to avoid. Just driving on a freeway entails risks, but you accept those risks to gain the benefit of rapid commuting. You are willing to accept the risks of air travel in exchange for the benefits of extraordinary speed and convenience. Even "little" decisions like whether or not to go skiing or even to play tennis require the acceptance of some degree of risk. Generally, the greater the *perceived* benefit, the more risk we are willing to take.

Evaluating risk/benefit ratios is part of every doctor's routine practice, and it's a major consideration in almost every decision we make in treating our patients. There are risks to every surgery or procedure we perform, every birth we attend and every medication we prescribe. We take that responsibility seriously, being ever mindful of our Hippocratic Oath in which we vow to "do no harm". Living up to that oath can be challenging, however, because absolutely nothing in the medical world is entirely risk-free. It wouldn't be reasonable, therefore, to assume that hormone replacement could be totally without risk.

ESTROGEN

I'll start with a discussion of estrogen, because of all the media attention this hormone has received and because it has been specifically identified as a potential health risk. Estrogen stimulates growth of the uterine lining, which can result in heavier or irregular bleeding. Unopposed estrogen is also known to increase the chance of uterine cancer. The significant word there is *unopposed*, meaning not balanced against proper levels of progesterone. (You may recall that one of the most important functions of progesterone is to counteract the negative effects of estrogen). We can eliminate this risk, however, by balancing those two hormones. A woman who has had a hysterectomy, of course, needn't consider that problem.

The possible effect of estrogen on the breast must be considered, however, partly because breast cancer is so common (whether a woman is using hormones or not), and because there's been so much publicity about the possible link between the two. You would think, with all of the attention that has been focused on that possible link, there would be a consensus opinion. Unfortunately, the data is still unclear and there is little agreement in the medical community as to the actual risk. In this abbreviated discussion, it's not possible to provide you with a detailed review of all the conflicting studies, but I will offer a short summary.

Some studies, performed by reputable researchers, show no difference in breast cancer incidence between women who use estrogen and those who do not. There are even studies that have shown an actual decrease in mortality from breast cancer in estrogen users. The study that generated the most publicity recently is the Women's Health Initiative that reported an increase of 8 breast cancers per year for every 10,000 women using a combination of a form of estrogen with a progestin. Even if that were the only finding in the study, the increase is quite low and the benefits might outweigh the small risk. However, that was not the only finding. The very same study also found that women who used hormones had a *reduced* risk of colon cancer that was about equal to the increase in risk for breast cancer. In other words, the *overall* risk of cancer was about the same for the women who took hormones as for those who didn't.

A much more important question is whether that study, which was conducted on women who were using synthetic estrogen and synthetic progestin, would have produced the same results if the women had been using bioidentical natural hormones. (I believe it would not have, and I am convinced that many of the negative effects occurred because artificial chemicals and improper doses were used.)

Other factors that may affect your use of estrogen are: age, medical history, family history, severity of symptoms and previous experience with hormones. Each of these is given careful consideration when I customize hormone replacement programs for my patients.

Having investigated the risk/benefit ratio thoroughly, I am convinced that the benefits of natural estrogen outweigh the risks for most women.

TESTOSTERONE

Testosterone raises much less concern because the risks associated with this hormone are relatively minor and easily managed, while the benefits (as detailed in an earlier chapter) are huge. In my experience, the most common side effects of testosterone—acne and unwanted hair growth—are rarely seen unless the dosages used are too high. That's why I monitor hormone levels so carefully in my patients and adjust the doses when necessary, before any side effects appear. In my opinion, the risk/benefit ratio of testosterone clearly favors its use.

THYROID

Thyroid can easily be monitored to avoid any significant side effects. Monitoring includes not only measurement of thyroid hormone levels in your blood, but also a careful assessment of any symptoms such as rapid heart rate. With careful observation of both, there is little risk that this hormone will cause you harm. The benefits, on the other hand, are numerous. Thyroid influences the function of every cell and organ in your body, and proper amounts are critical to your health.

PREGNENOLONE

Pregnenolone, known primarily as a precursor of other hormones, has also been shown to enhance brain function, memory and mood. This hormone has no adverse effects, so you can take advantage of its benefits without risk. In fact, since pregnenolone is a food derivative, it is not even controlled by the FDA. For this particular hormone, risk/benefit ratio certainly favors its use.

DHEA

DHEA is another hormone that is available over the counter (without a prescription). DHEA is well tolerated even in very high doses, but because it is a precursor to testosterone, high doses have been associated with acne and unwanted hair growth. This side effect can be avoided by lowering the dosage. In my opinion, the benefits of DHEA outweigh the risks.

HGH

The risk/benefit analysis is less clear for HGH. In spite of numerous research studies and ample evidence of its benefits, the general medical community has limited experience with its use. After carefully studying the available literature and observing patients for several years while they used HGH, I have encountered only minor problems that are easily managed. There is no evidence that HGH causes cancer or any other serious medical problem. Unfortunately, there is also no strong evidence that it has the miraculous power to keep you forever young or rejuvenate the near-dead. Nonetheless, I believe that HGH promotes healing, helps slow the aging process, and provides the many benefits detailed previously. Therefore, I recommend it to my patients and I use it myself. Because HGH is so expensive, some of my patients choose not to include it in their natural hormone replacement program. I accept their decision, but wish for their sake that finances weren't a barrier.

*   *   *

If, after reading this book, you still have questions about hormone risks and benefits, I urge you to review other sources. There is an abundance of information available about each of these hormones on the internet and every bookstore has numerous books on all aspects of this subject. Be prepared, however, to find a variety of contradictory facts and conflicting opinions about hormone use. The frustrating reality is that many medical questions still cannot be answered simply or unanimously.

In my experience, the potential benefits of natural hormone

replacement significantly outweigh the potential risks for most women. Every woman is different, and each woman must make the decision for herself. You know best which benefits are important to you and which risks you are willing to take. It's *your* quality of life, so as I said in my short answer above, you get to make the final decision.

X.

DO MEN NEED HORMONES?

Q: *Do men need hormones?*

A: *Yes. As men age they become deficient in five essential hormones.*

Until recently, hormone therapy has been primarily a women's health issue. Hormone replacement therapy for men was never a concern for me, since I am a gynecologist, and my practice was limited to treating women. Things changed dramatically, however, when I began to focus on natural hormone replacement and started meeting the husbands of my patients. These men often accompanied their wives to my office for consultations, and they attended my lectures and workshops, which were designed for women.

At first, the men just listened quietly, but it was not long before they started asking questions themselves. They, too, were troubled by changes they noticed in themselves as they grew older, and they were eager to know if hormone replacement could do as much for them as for their wives. The answer is yes. Men can definitely alter the course of deterioration that would otherwise follow the declining hormone levels that accompany aging.

The loss of men's hormones has been called "andropause". It has not generated as much attention in men as menopause has in women because the hormonal decline in men is more gradual, and the symptoms—at least in the beginning—are more subtle. In menopause, the abrupt changes cause such marked symptoms that women are motivated to seek relief.

Men and women are far less knowledgeable about andropause than about menopause, and only recently have men been willing to even consider help. (That is not surprising, since men have never been as likely as women to seek medical care unless they have an injury or serious illness.) An even greater obstacle when it comes to hormones is that men may perceive the need to replace hormones as a challenge to their masculinity. (*Real* men aren't supposed to admit weakness.)

Male hormone levels begin to decline as early as the mid-twenties, but the consequences are not usually noticeable until a man is in his forties. From that time on, the hormone decline accelerates along with the symptoms.

The five hormones essential to a man's well being are: testosterone, DHEA, thyroid, pregnenolone and HGH. While the levels of all will decline, *testosterone* is the hormone that a man is most likely to consider important. He is not alone in appreciating the importance of testosterone. The researchers who isolated and synthesized testosterone were awarded the Nobel Prize for their work.

The two most common and prominent symptoms of hormone loss in men are both related to diminished testosterone: muscle loss (which typically appears first) and decreased sex drive and performance.

Without exception, men notice a change in their muscles and body shape as they age. Their muscles become smaller and softer, and waistlines expand. The midsection growth is due partly to increasing fat deposition between the abdominal muscles and skin, and partly to fat inside the abdominal wall known as "visceral fat". At this stage of life, no matter how many hours a man spends in the gym, his muscles just won't grow and he can't create the same muscular "definition" that was possible in his youth. In fact, those goals simply aren't achievable unless testosterone is returned to its youthful level. HGH and thyroid hormone will probably also need to be supplemented. It's not just a cosmetic issue: the increased visceral fat is a sign of increased risk for cardio-vascular disease and type II diabetes.

Testosterone levels continue to drop slowly after age 40, and by the age of 60, sixty percent of men have measurably low levels that are linked directly to decreased sex drive and performance. Men view their loss of desire for sex and their declining ability to perform as direct insults to their masculinity and virility. However, it is an absolute fact of life that, with age, a man's erections are not as frequent, as firm or as lasting. Nonetheless, men who experience these changes have been very reluctant to seek advice or treatment. You could hear a collective sigh of relief across this nation when men observed the explosive popularity of Viagra. Suddenly, men of all ages were using a pill to enhance erections. This was clear evidence that the problem was universal, and that men could now accept treatment for it without embarrassment.

Ironically, it's misleading to judge a man's hormone health solely on his ability to have an erection, since that may be the last thing to go. In fact, testosterone levels may drop significantly long before that point is reached. Restoring testosterone to healthy levels may not only help prevent erectile dysfunction, but provides all of the other benefits I've mentioned earlier.

I have already discussed the benefits of increased strength and endurance provided by testosterone. Prevention of bone loss is another. Although osteoporosis occurs more commonly in women, men are also victims of bone loss and osteoporosis. As men live to older age and testosterone levels fall, bone fractures increase in frequency, and weakness of the vertebral bones leads to their collapse and to shrinking height. (Many of us have been surprised and shocked to notice that our fathers—who used to be taller than we were—became shorter.) Collapse of the vertebrae also causes back pain and sciatic nerve problems.

Finally, it's important to note that testosterone also improves heart health by decreasing total cholesterol levels while maintaining levels of HDL (the "good" cholesterol), and by dilating coronary arteries, which increases blood flow to the heart muscle.

I can't leave the topic of testosterone without addressing concerns about its possible effect on the health of the prostate gland. I will start by stating that in spite of considerable controversy over the association of testosterone with prostate health, there is no evidence that testosterone causes prostate cancer. There is some concern, however, that it may stimulate cell growth of an existing cancer. It is therefore imperative that any man considering its use first have all appropriate tests to screen for prostate health. This would include at least an annual physical exam plus specific blood tests that could detect prostate disease. It is interesting to note that the incidence of prostate cancer actually increases as levels of testosterone decrease. Young men with the highest levels of testosterone have the lowest incidence of prostate cancer. Nevertheless, as men live longer, they must be increasingly vigilant, because prostate cancer is a very insidious disease and can remain silent for many years.

DHEA is another hormone that men need to replace as they age. By age 50, men produce only half as much DHEA as they did at age 25 and the decline continues with time. A deficiency of DHEA is associated with fatigue, lack of stamina, memory loss, dry skin and poor sex drive. The body's immune system is also weakened as DHEA diminishes, due to the important role this hormone plays in maintaining immune strength. Supplementation with DHEA counters all of the above problems, as well as improving sleep and increasing energy.

Pregnenolone plays an important supporting role in the body's physiology. It is particularly beneficial in brain cell repair and brain function. Pregnenolone is a potent memory enhancer, and contributes to intelligence, learning ability, alertness and the feeling of well-being. It is also considered an anti-stress hormone. Because it is a precursor to other hormones, as pregnenolone declines, so does production of those hormones.

Thyroid is the hormone that is responsible for regulating body metabolism, temperature and certain cerebral functions. This hormone often declines with age, leading to weight gain, fatigue, depression, sleep disturbances, dry skin, thin hair and forgetfulness. All of these symptoms are readily relieved by replacing thyroid to its optimum level. Thyroid hormone also increases fat breakdown in the body and reduces blood cholesterol levels.

HGH is the fifth essential hormone that is likely to be deficient. HGH is known as the healing hormone because of its ability to stimulate cell growth and rejuvenation. Like other hormones, HGH peaks in our early 20's and has dropped to half that peak amount by 50. HGH has been shown to increase lean muscle mass while decreasing visceral fat (the fat that accumulates inside the abdomen which is largely responsible for the expanding waist lines that are so difficult to reduce). Signs of HGH deficiency include: thin, inelastic skin; high body fat; elevated cholesterol; poor muscle tone; poor exercise endurance; bone density loss; thinning hair and poor sleep. Benefits of correcting a deficiency in this hormone are seen over a longer period of time than the more quickly appreciated benefits of thyroid.

In summary, men are likely to become deficient in five essential hormones as they age: testosterone, DHEA, thyroid, pregnenolone and HGH. All of these hormones have important and vital functions in maintaining a man's health. Conversely, a deficiency of any one can cause symptoms and signs of aging. Initial symptoms are subtle and often ignored by men until damage has already taken place. Because prevention is more effective than repair, men should be encouraged to have their hormone levels tested early and to replace hormones to optimum levels before any damage takes place.

.

XI.

ARE HORMONES ENOUGH?

Q: *Are hormones enough?*
A: *No. They are essential, but they can't do it alone.*

I wish I could promise that you could achieve eternal youth and health just by maintaining optimum hormone levels. It's not that simple. Good health does require the presence and balance of the hormones I've discussed, but other factors must be considered. If you are serious about protecting yourself against the signs and symptoms of aging, you'll have to give those hormones some help in doing their jobs.

In previous pages, I've described how testosterone and HGH help build lean muscle mass and reduce the ratio of fat to muscle in your body. I've shown you how estrogen, progesterone and testosterone increase bone strength and defend you against osteoporosis. None of this can happen without physical activity. (Please note that I purposely didn't say "exercise", because that term has a negative connotation in some people's minds.) Any kind of physical activity will support the beneficial effects of these hormones. If working out in a gym doesn't appeal to you, there are many other options that will work very well.

Your body is just as invigorated, energized and strengthened by walking briskly to and from the store as it is by running on a computerized treadmill. Working in your garden is as good for your back, shoulders, arms and legs as using Nautilus equipment in the gym. Doing deep breathing exercises while watching TV will give you many of the same benefits as deep breathing through aerobic exercise.

This is not intended to discourage you from participating in formal exercise or training programs. If you enjoy working out in a gym or participating in yoga or Pilates classes, I encourage you to do it as often as possible. I also advocate the use of free weights for targeting specific muscle groups, because that will not only strengthen muscles and bones, but can sculpt and shape your body. Sports such as swimming, riding bikes, hiking and tennis are also excellent physical activities.

Your body is uniquely engineered, so using your muscles and bones actually builds them up rather than wearing them down. Any activity, therefore, is beneficial as long as it isn't excessive and doesn't cause injury. My advice is to choose the activities that you like to do and that best suit your lifestyle. Then do them as often and as vigorously as you comfortably can. The important thing to remember is that you *must* keep your body moving to remain healthy and youthful.

You should also make a conscious effort to maintain or, if necessary, reduce your weight. If, at the age of 40, you continue to eat the same as when you were 20, you will automatically gain weight. This happens because your metabolism slows as you age, so you burn fewer calories every day. Over the course of a year, it can add three to five pounds to your weight. You can just imagine what those pounds do to the shape of your waist, hips and thighs—especially if you add the extra pounds year after year.

Balancing hormones can only do so much towards stimulating metabolism and protecting against excessive fat storage. You must do your part by reducing caloric input. I don't like the word "diet" because that has come to mean a short-term program of restricted food choices, and that is not what I have in mind. Although diets may be effective for losing weight, the lost weight is almost always regained. The alternative, which is far better, is to change your eating habits.

The simple (and perhaps sad) fact is that to be healthy, you have to eat less food. The type of food is much less important than the quantity. Eating too much "good" food is still bad for you, and most of the "bad" foods you have been warned about are perfectly fine if consumed in reasonable amounts.

I wrote earlier about the signals your body is constantly sending to maintain physiologic balance. One of those signals—when your body needs fuel—is the sensation of hunger. An equally important signal to watch for is the one that says you are no longer hungry. If you ignore that one you will consume more food than your body has requested and you will gain weight. The best way to keep your weight in check is simply to eat only when you are hungry. As obvious as that advice sounds, it is difficult to follow because we all eat for many other reasons: to be sociable; to be courteous; to enjoy certain tastes; to reward ourselves; to comfort ourselves and even to avoid waste.

Another important reason why we eat more than we really need is the delay that exists between the time when we eat and when the body stops sending its hunger signals. Pausing for short breaks during meals will help you overcome that problem, and prevent that uncomfortable, overstuffed feeling that comes from eating too much, too fast.

In your quest to avoid gaining weight, I don't suggest that you deprive yourself of foods that you particularly enjoy, even if they are "fattening". When we deprive ourselves of something we truly love, we are inclined to reward ourselves later for having been good. That "reward" may be more fattening than what we gave up in the first place.

The bottom line, no matter what else you may have heard, is that you only gain weight if you consume more calories than you use up. That is more likely to happen as you age, unless you adjust for changes in your metabolism and activity. Even if your hormones are adequate, once you reach your ideal adult weight, staying there usually requires that you steadily decrease your consumption of food. Research shows that low caloric intake is good for your health. In fact, it may be one of the key factors in increasing longevity. Stop listening to the "experts" who tell you how many ounces of which foods you should eat at what time of day. Start listening instead to your body, which will give you much more important information. And remember, food, like so many other things in life, is best enjoyed in moderation.

Stress is another important area that should be addressed, because your health is negatively affected by stress, and yet there is no way to avoid it entirely. To maintain good health, your only option is to find healthy ways to deal with stress.

Several hormones, especially estrogen, DHEA and pregnenolone, are known to be helpful, but there are a number of other powerful stress-relievers you can—and should—consider before resorting to your medicine cabinet. Methods range from something as simple as breathing exercises that can be done anytime, anywhere, to sophisticated measures like biofeedback training. Strolling on the beach or in the park, which doesn't take any training, can be very effective.

Yoga can take you to deeper and more profound levels of relaxation than a warm bath, candles and soothing music. However, if you don't have the time or inclination to learn and practice yoga, but are willing to soak in a tub at the end of the day while listening to music in a candle-lit room, then that might be a better method for *you*.

Laughter is another wonderful stress reliever. It has not only been shown to relieve stress, but has been proven to actually improve your immune system strength and create a clearer mind. Laughter makes us all feel better, and nothing, after all, is more important than that. Which method you select for relieving the stress in your life is not important. It is important, though, to find *some* ways to combat stress in order to keep it from damaging your health.

Finally, although I'm probably stating the obvious, I feel obligated to remind you that hormone replacement is medical treatment that should not be started before your health has been thoroughly evaluated with appropriate screening tests. (These actually aren't additional tests, but the ones you should already be getting as part of your routine health care.) Your annual examinations should include pap smears, mammograms, and blood tests that are specifically appropriate for your age and medical history. Periodically, depending on your age, additional tests such as EKGs, bone density scans and colonoscopies should also be performed.

In addition to the routine physical exams, blood tests, EKGs and colonoscopies described above, men also require regular prostate screening, which includes the measurement of blood PSA levels.

As essential as hormones are, they can't do it alone. Even if you keep all hormones at their optimum levels, it is still important to get regular physical activity, eat sensibly, find time to relax and pay attention to your other health needs.

XII.

WHAT IS THE NEXT STEP?

Q: *What is the next step?*

A: *Schedule a consultation with a physician who specializes in the use of natural hormones.*

If you are considering the use of natural hormones, I strongly recommend that you consult a physician who specializes in their use. I'll explain why your choice of physician is important.

Hormone replacement differs significantly from standard drug treatment for disease, because—with hormones—one size does *not* fit all. To get the maximum benefits from hormone replacement, the prescription for each hormone must be customized to meet *your* unique needs and adjusted frequently. That's different from the way doctors treat many diseases, where a standard dose of medication can be used. (For example, when treating an infection, most adults can be given essentially the same prescription.)

Many factors must be taken into consideration in determining your particular hormone replacement needs, starting with your age. Since production of hormones by your glands declines with age, if you begin therapy in your 40's, your hormone requirements will clearly be different from what they will be if you start in your 60's. The presence or absence of symptoms from hormone deficiency is another important factor to be considered, along with your size, body type, lifestyle and genetic background. Your pre-treatment hormone levels (as measured by blood tests) are also used to determine your initial hormone doses.

Once your replacement program has started, it is important to measure hormone levels in your blood at regular intervals and to monitor your response to therapy. Your ongoing requirement for replacement hormones may be affected by hormones from your own endocrine glands which—though less efficient than at their peak—may still be active. Since the amount of that hormone being produced varies, it is often necessary to adjust replacement hormones. Periodic monitoring is also required because your own needs do not remain constant. Over time, they will be altered by your body's natural changes and by its response to the replacement hormones you are using.

These and other factors make it necessary for your physician to devote a considerable amount of time to assessing your hormone needs, designing a supplement program for you, and monitoring your therapy. Done properly, this is quite labor-intensive. It is this need to customize that discourages some physicians from utilizing natural hormone therapy, because it takes much more time and attention than writing standard prescriptions. Many physicians can not, or are not willing to devote the requisite amount time to a specialty service such as this.

Those of us who truly appreciate the benefits available through use of natural hormones are willing to spend the time and effort necessary to make those benefits available to our patients. I do this because I believe that hormone therapy is much more than a temporary way to relieve menopausal symptoms. I believe it is an essential component of long-term total health care. I also recognize that in order for you to benefit most, we must work closely together to determine the correct dose of each hormone, not only at the start of therapy, but for as long as hormone replacement continues. This means that if you ask me to assume responsibility for your hormone replacement, we will see a lot of each other—especially over the first year.

Our initial consultation begins with an in-depth review of your medical history and a discussion of your past or current symptoms. Then, I'll answer your questions, and order appropriate laboratory tests to measure your pre-treatment hormone levels. When the lab results have been reviewed, and after taking all of the above factors into consideration, a natural hormone replacement program is customized to meet your specific needs. I will prescribe the amount of each hormone that I believe is needed for your optimum health.

Over the next several weeks, we will speak frequently as I monitor your progress and answer any questions that might arise. About two months after the initial visit, we will meet again in the office for a progress update and to draw blood for follow-up laboratory tests. Once the results of those tests are reviewed, prescriptions will be adjusted as necessary. For the following three months, we stay in touch, usually by phone, to discuss any changes in your symptoms and to determine if any adjustments in the hormone prescriptions are necessary.

At approximately six months, another office consultation is scheduled and a third set of blood tests is done. Based upon those results, and on how you feel and look, other adjustments might be made. For the remainder of that first year, hormone prescriptions will probably remain fairly stable, although I will continue to monitor your progress. At the start of the second year, a complete re-evaluation is in order.

That is a brief outline of how your natural hormone replacement program would be managed in my office. It is important to remember that the entire process is only a part of—not a substitute for—your routine health screening and care as detailed in the previous chapter.

Over the course of the first year, you should notice several improvements in the way you look and feel. Energy levels and libido increase quickly when low levels of thyroid and testosterone are corrected. Most patients report improved skin quality early in the program. Menopausal symptoms are very responsive. Those who have had a problem with their weight are often surprised by their new success in dropping excess pounds. Weight loss, muscle tone and body fat all respond well to hormone replacement, but all depend to a great extent on your physical activity and caloric intake.

The more deficient in hormones you are at the outset, the more dramatic the results are likely to be. All of your individual responses will, of course, also depend upon your age, health and hormone status at the start of the program.

There is no "quick-fix" for aging and it can't be cured! If you decide to embark on this program, it should be with the understanding that it will be a long-term commitment, with rewards that justify the effort.

Your next step is simply to schedule a consultation.

A FINAL THOUGHT

This book was written to help you understand and appreciate the value of Natural Hormone Replacement. I hope it has motivated you to take advantage of the many benefits it offers. You live by a different set of standards than those of your grandmother, and you expect more from life. She didn't expect to be youthful, vivacious and beautiful at age 60, but you do—and should. She didn't have your high expectations or the means to accomplish them.

Fortunately, times have changed and it is no longer necessary to wait helplessly while the aging process slowly robs you of your youth and health. You can choose to defend against that process and enjoy more years of health, vitality, beauty and sexuality.

A growing number of physicians recognize the value of this therapy and have incorporated it into their practices, as I have. I encourage you to take the next step, schedule a consultation with one who specializes in this exciting new field and determine if this therapy is appropriate for you.